I'm Getting New Bifocals!

A Parody for Grown-Ups

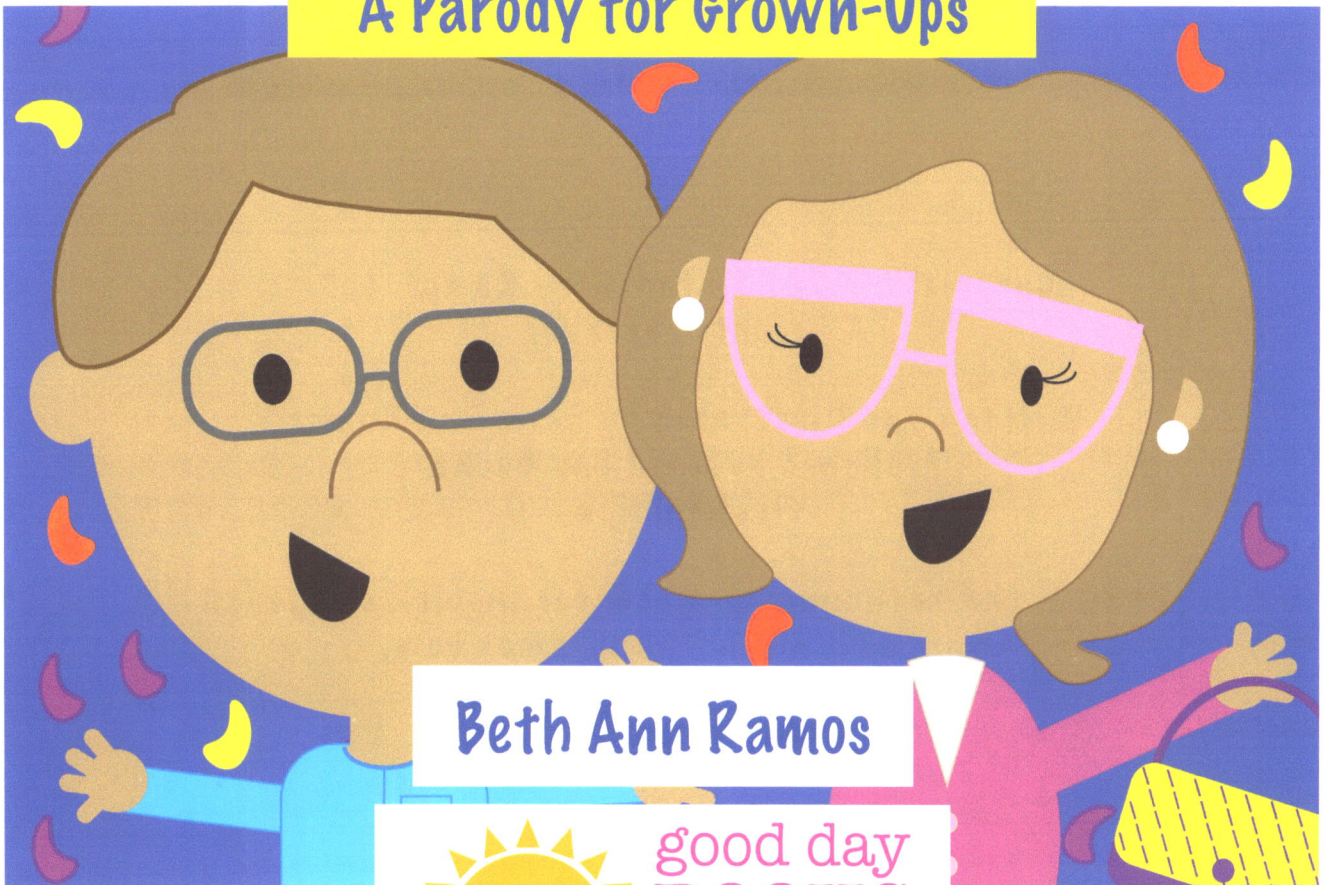

Beth Ann Ramos

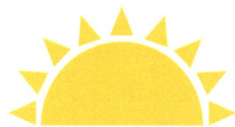

good day BOOKS

For:

_____

You look great in your new bifocals!

Written and Illustrated by Beth Ann Ramos
Published by Good Day Books
First Edition

Email beth@bethannramos.com for inquiries or learn
more at www.bethannramos.com.

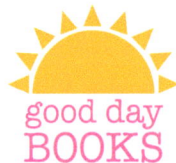

good day
BOOKS

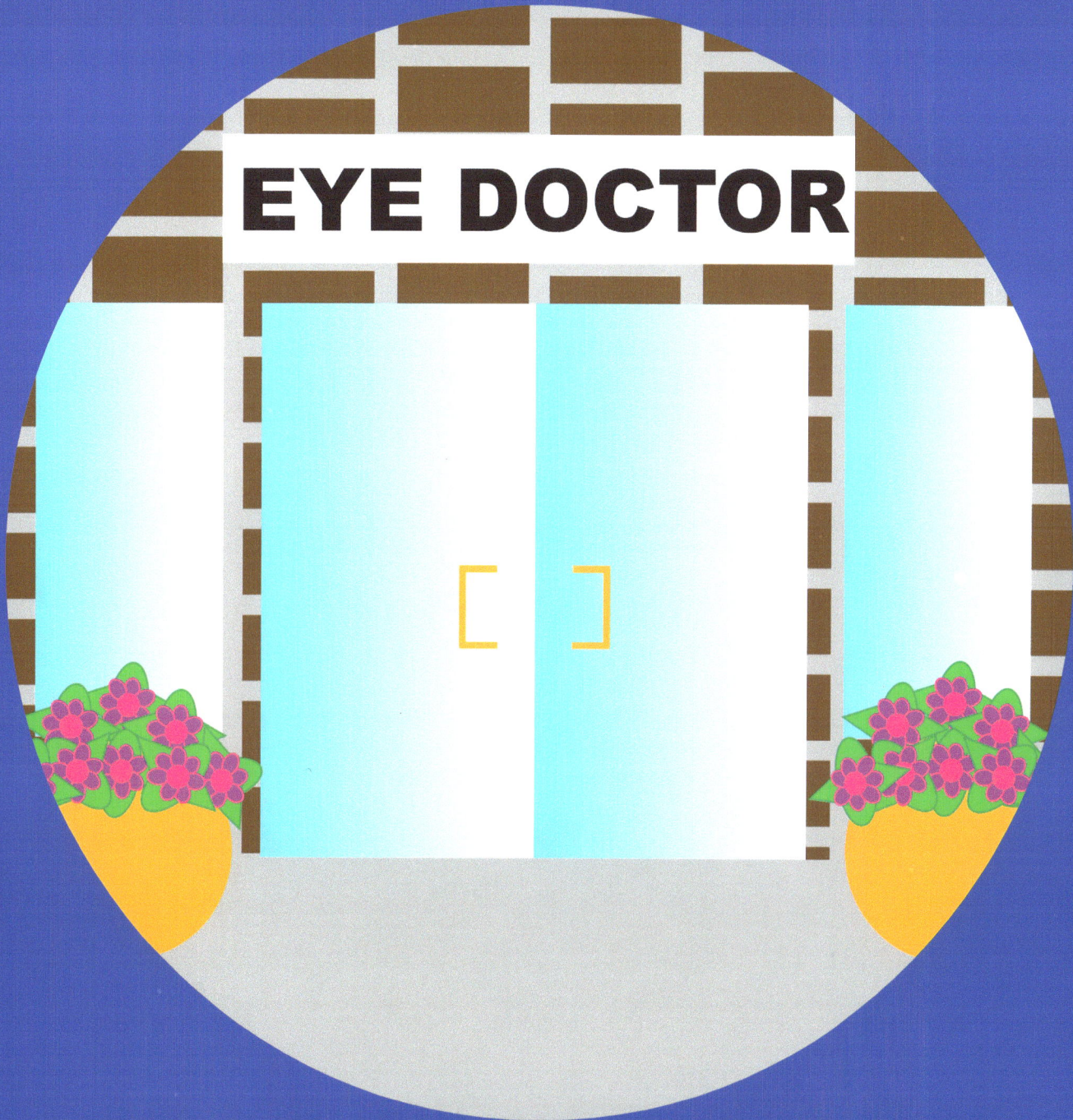

I'm getting new bifocals
so I can see...

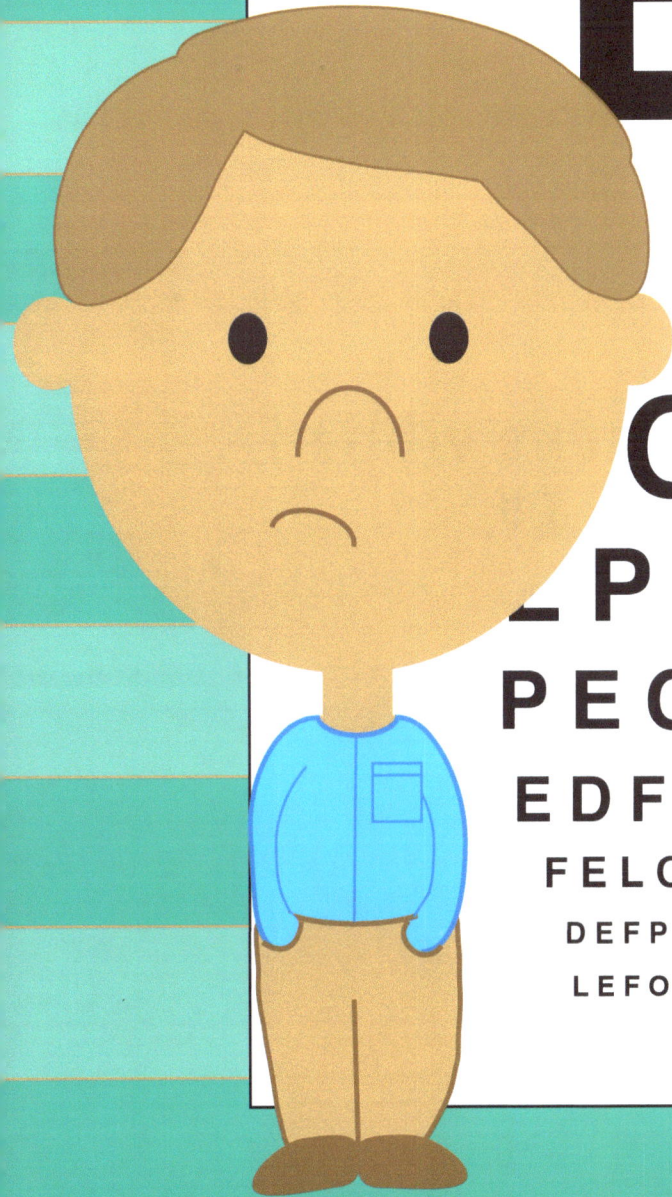

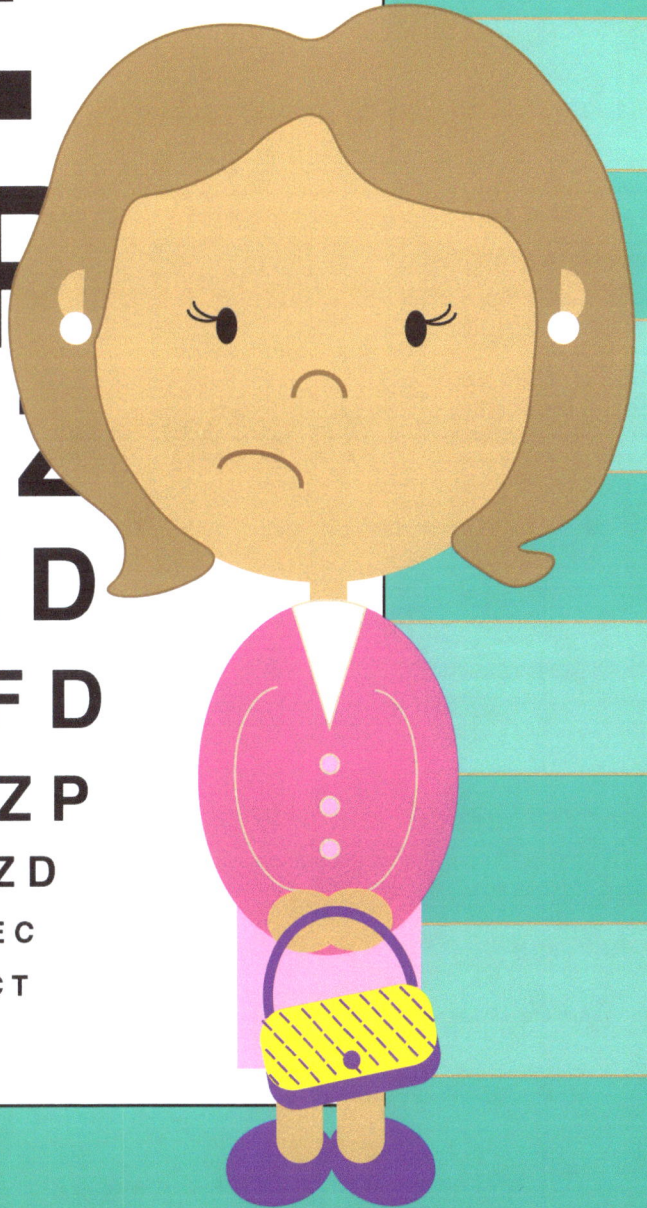

To play on my phone while I watch the TV.

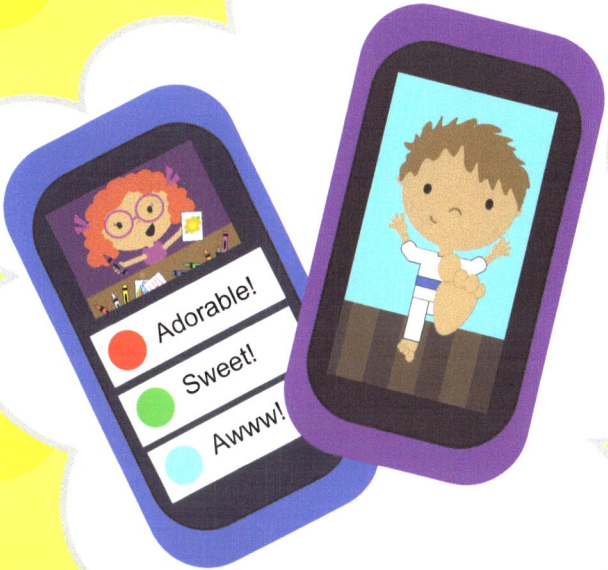

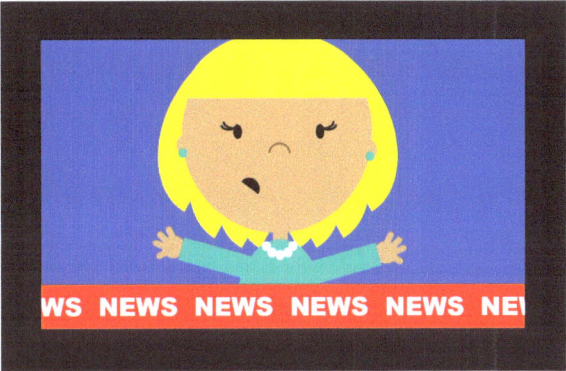

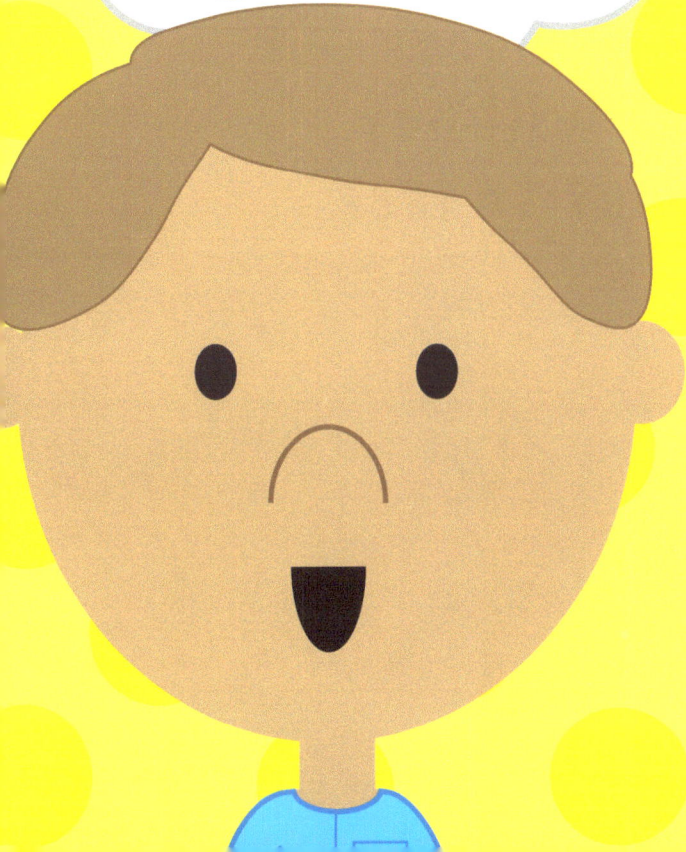

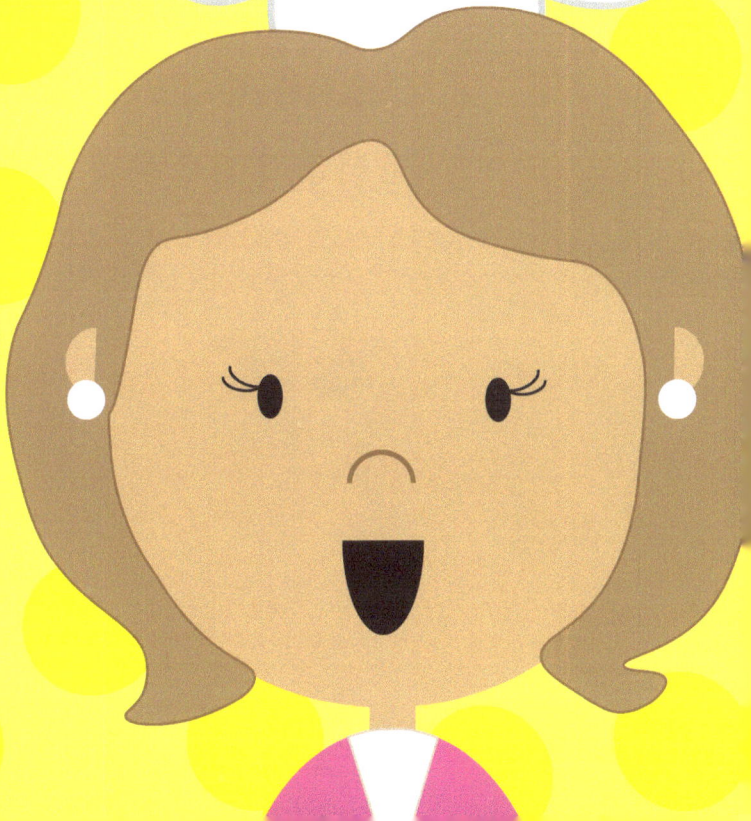

Which pair will I pick?
I'm excited to choose
some frames I will buy
and then try not to lose.

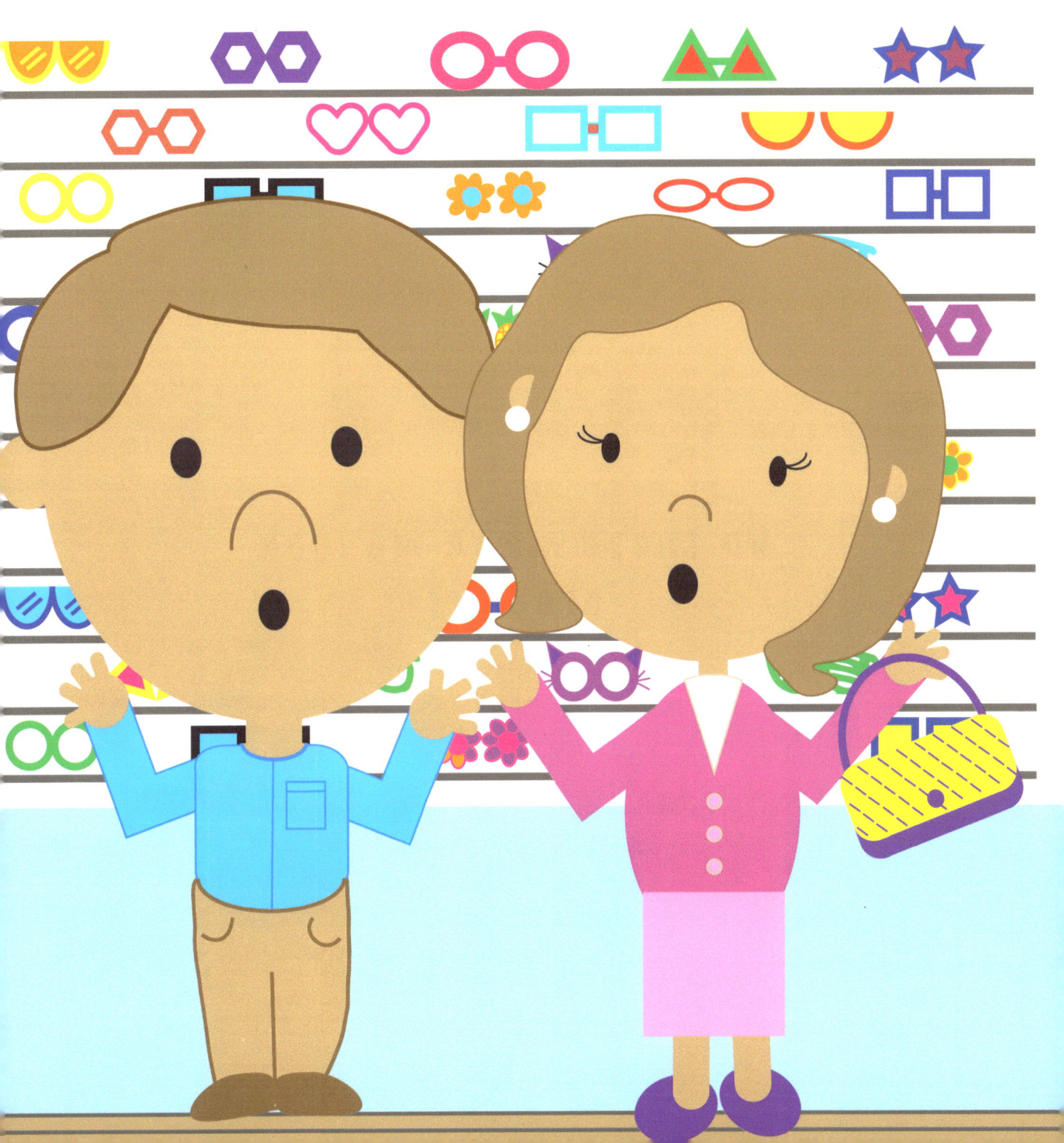

Do these make me look groovy?

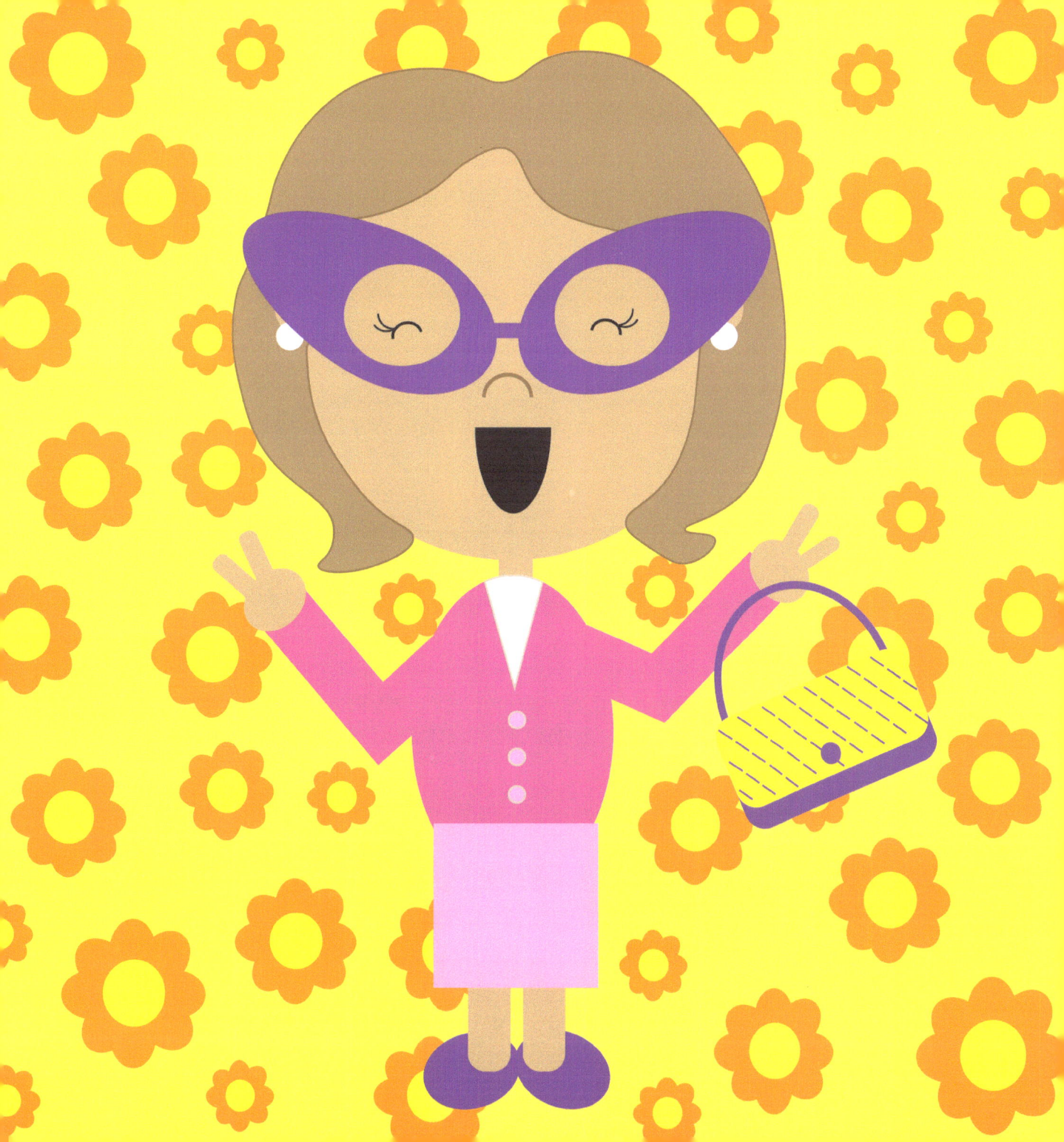

Or better?
Or worse?

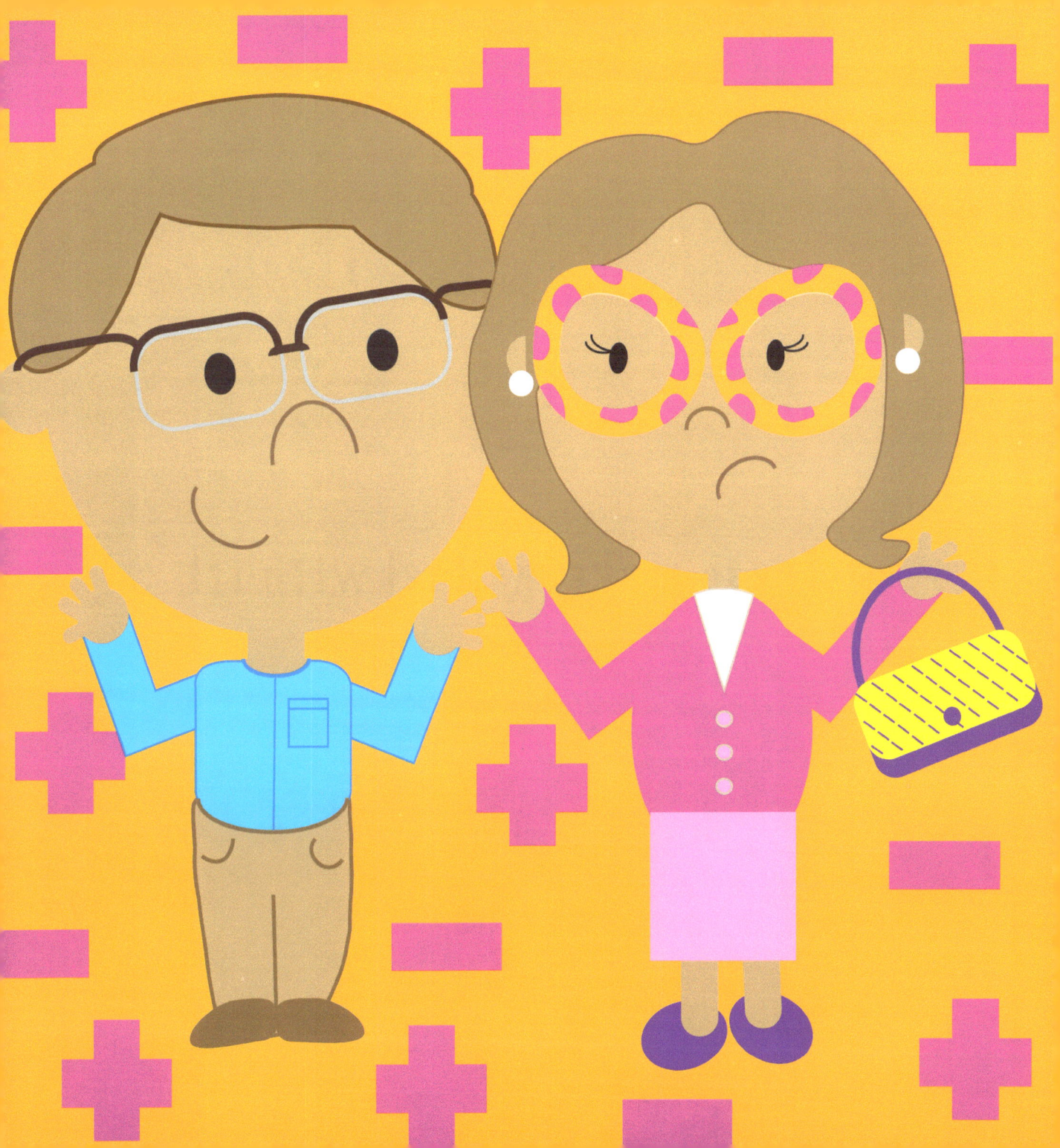

These make me feel with it!

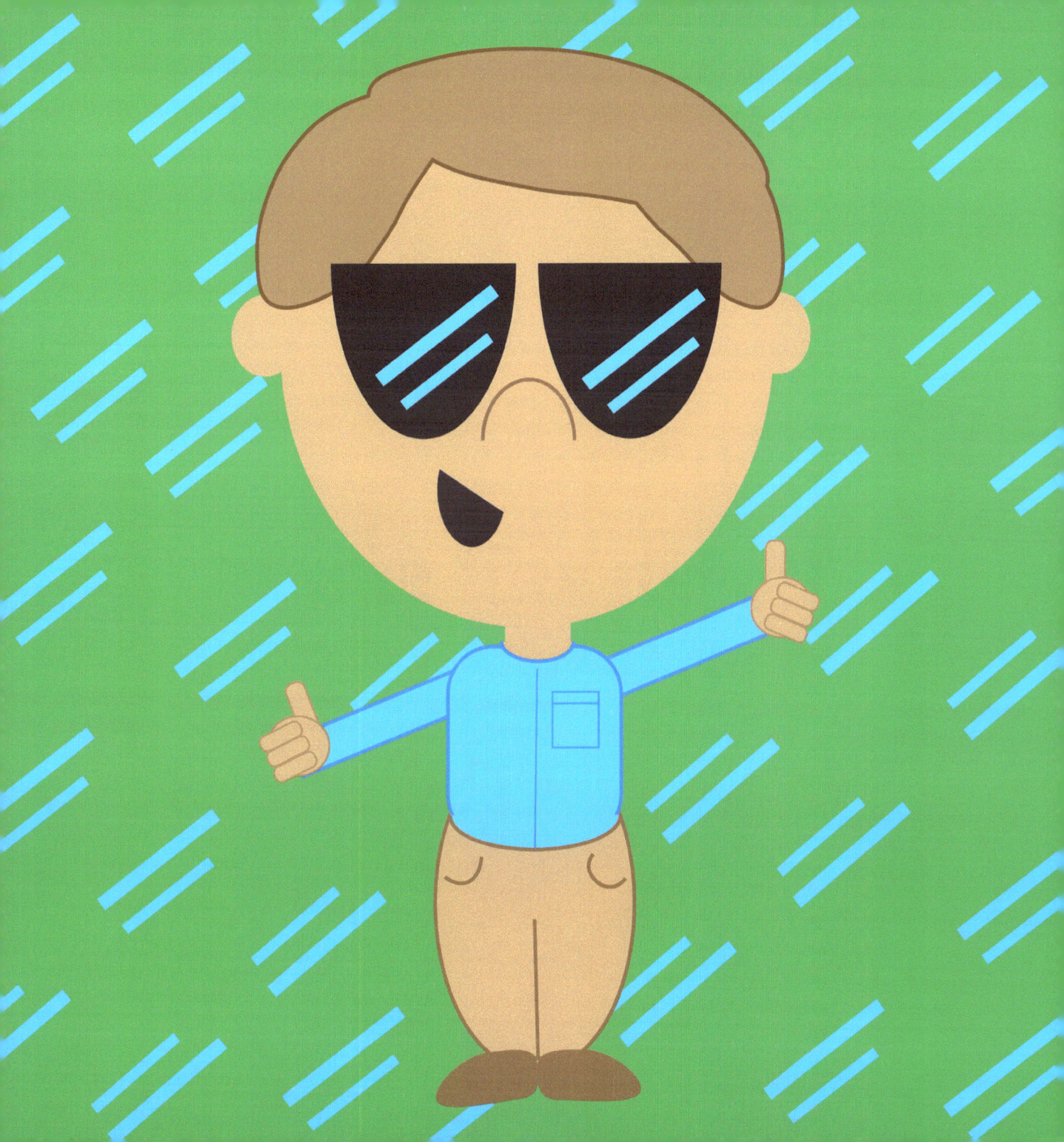

But these match my purse!

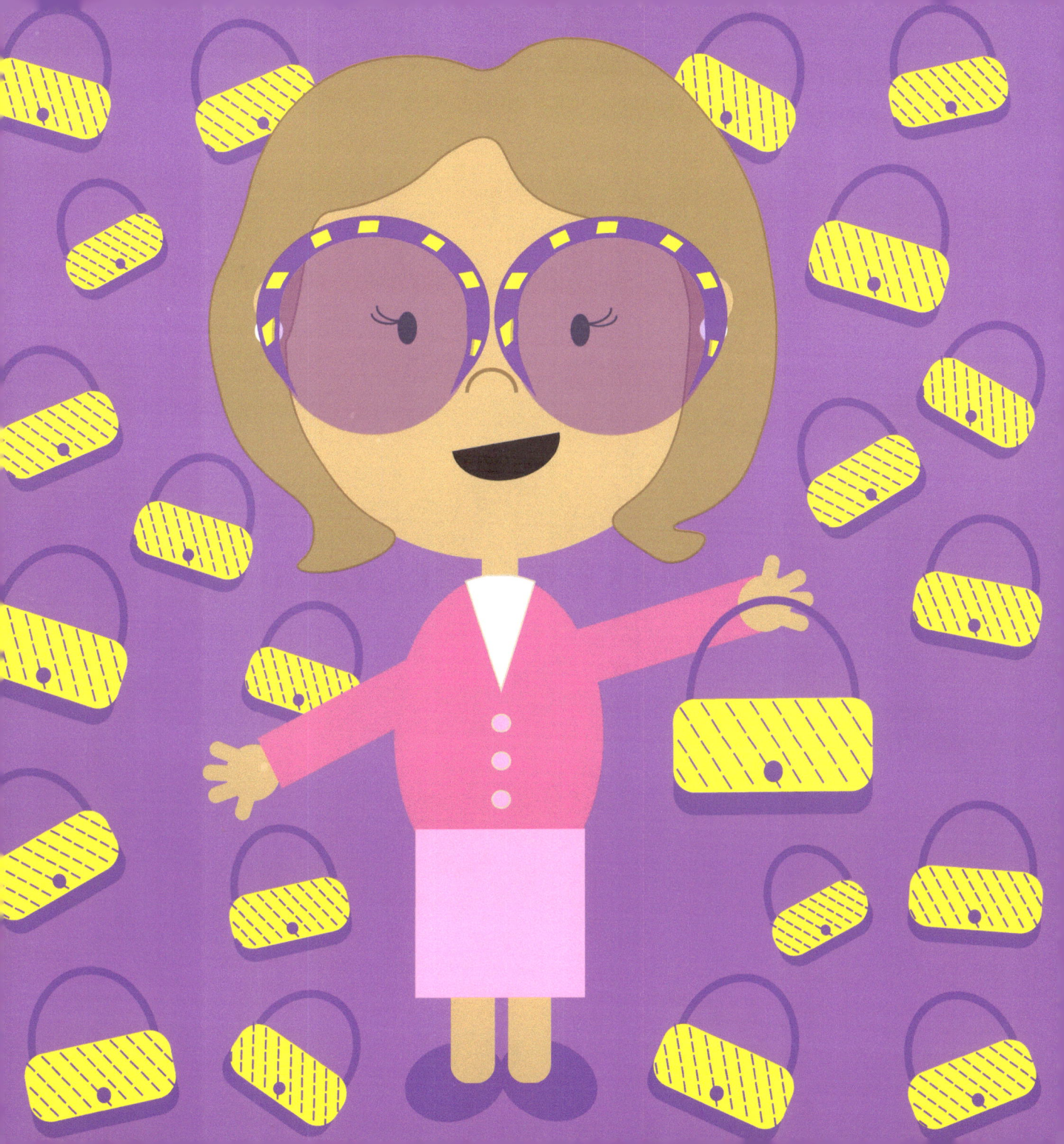

These make me feel dashing!

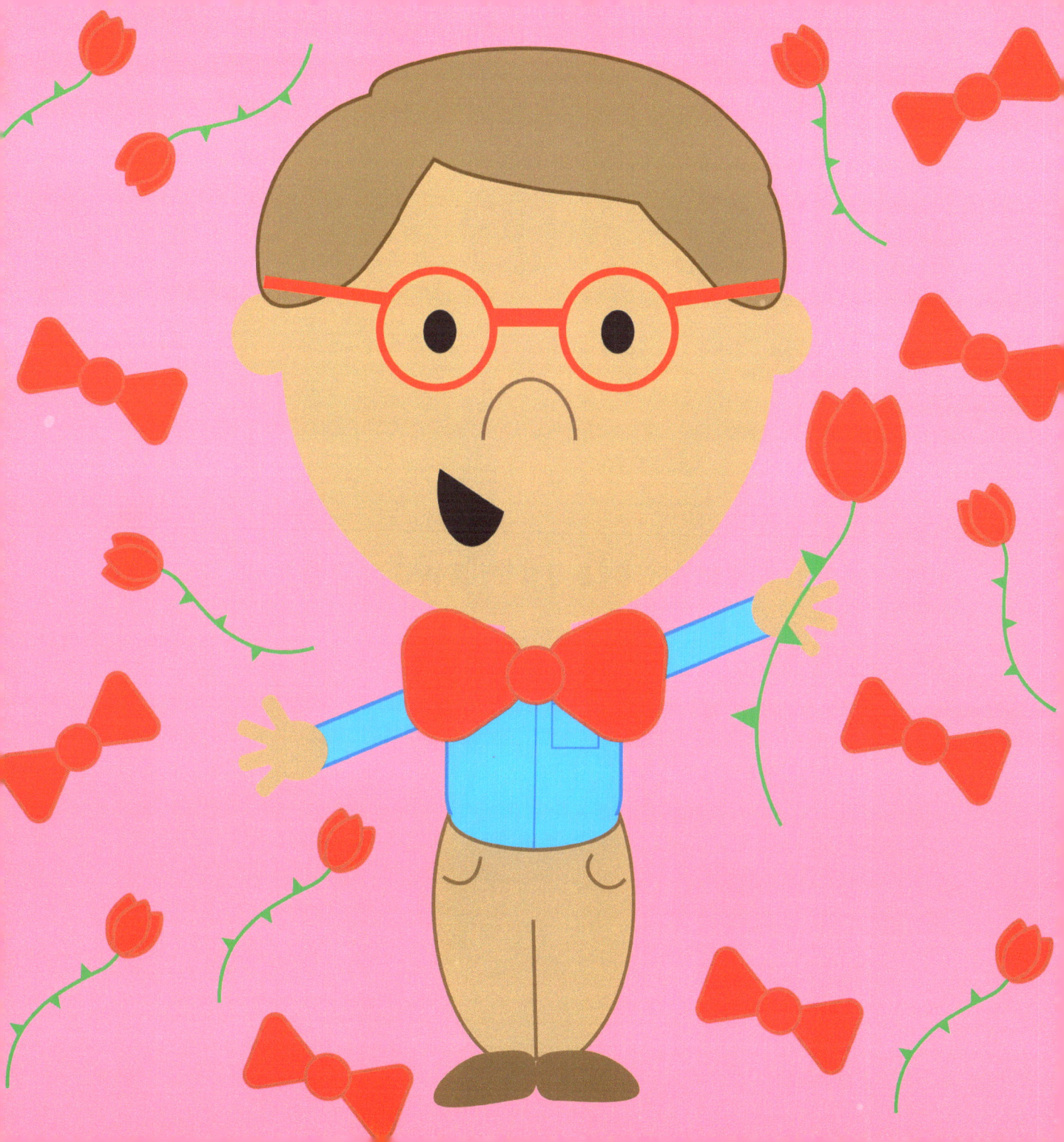

Now, classy and rad!

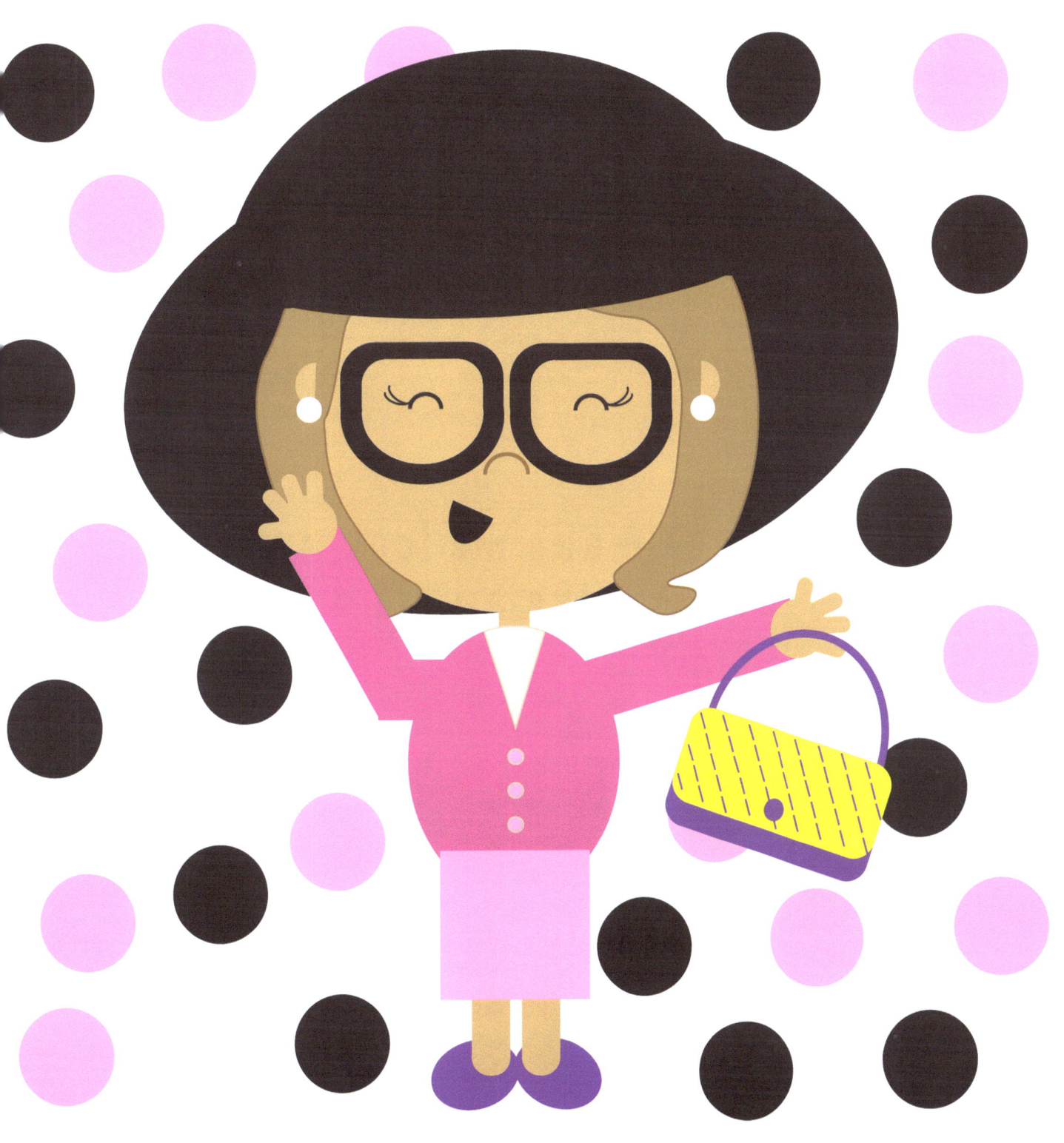

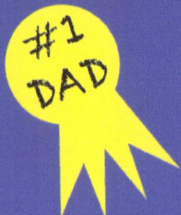

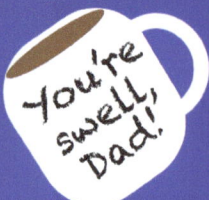

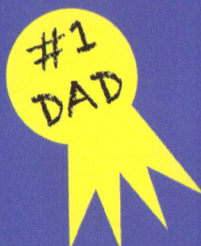

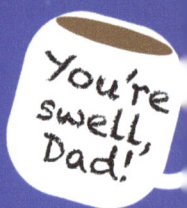

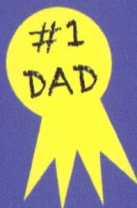

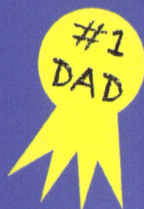

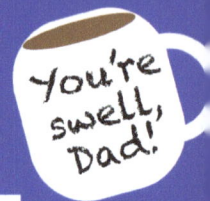

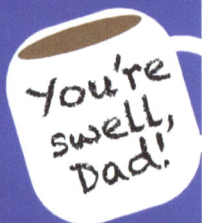

Do these make me look swell?
Or just like an old dad?

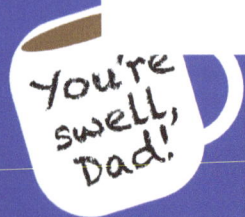

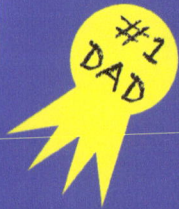

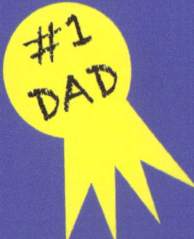

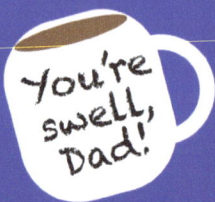

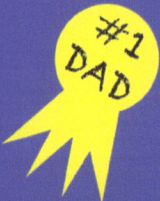

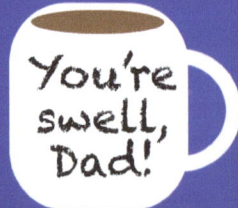

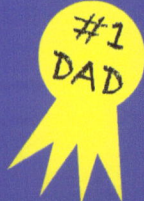

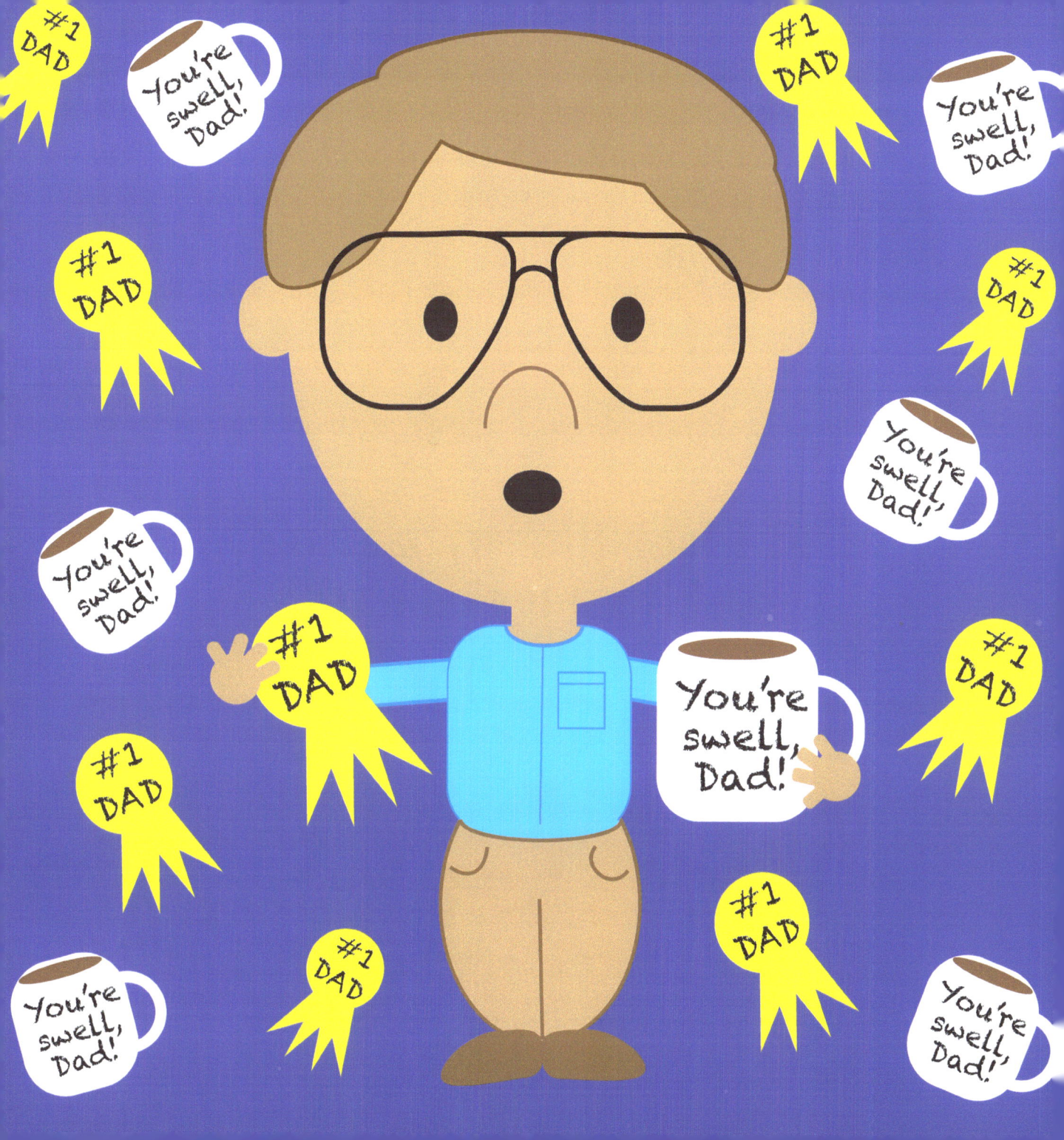

Do I look like my mother?
I think I look smart!

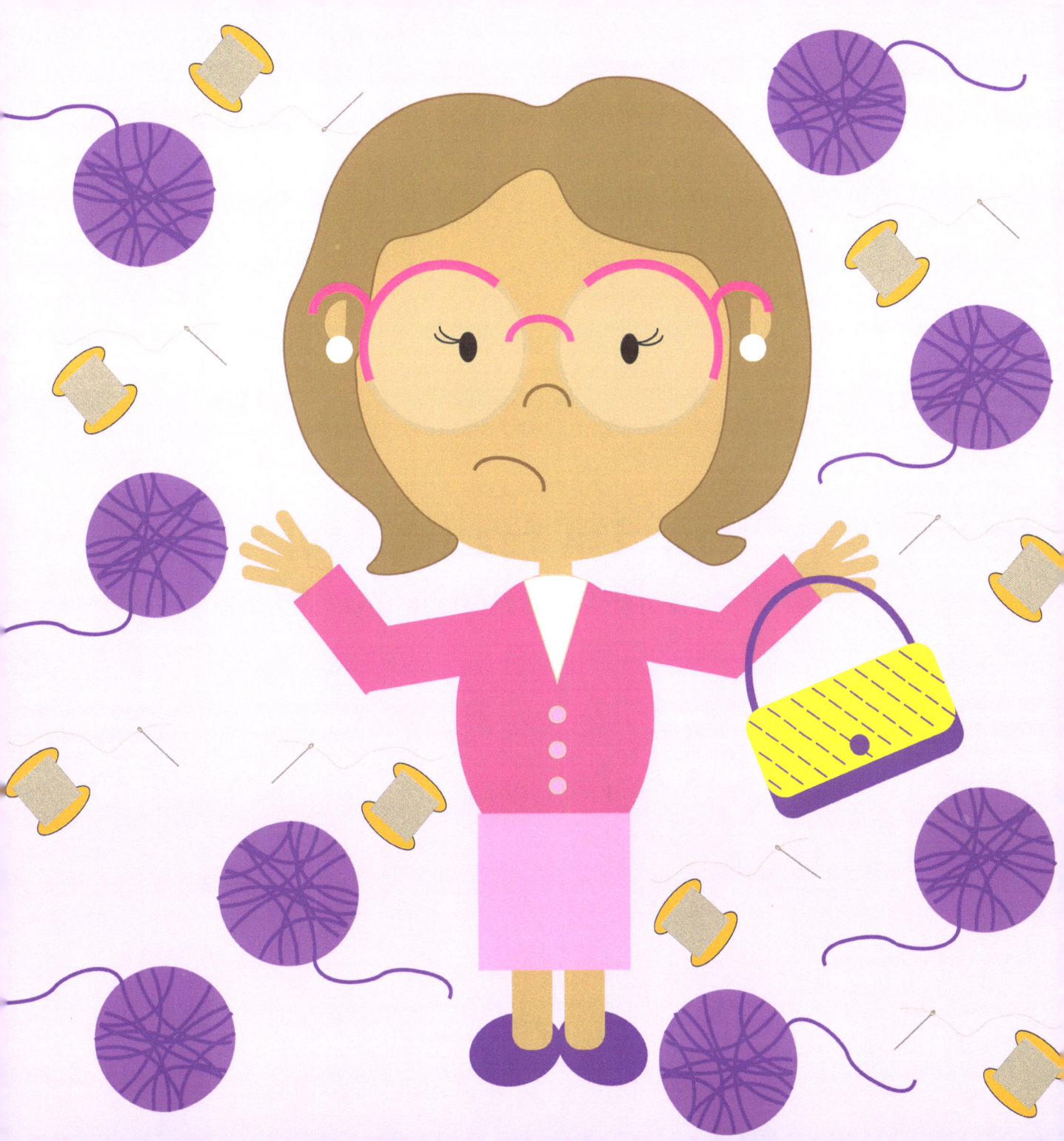

Now, I'm feeling hip!
Am I just an old fart?

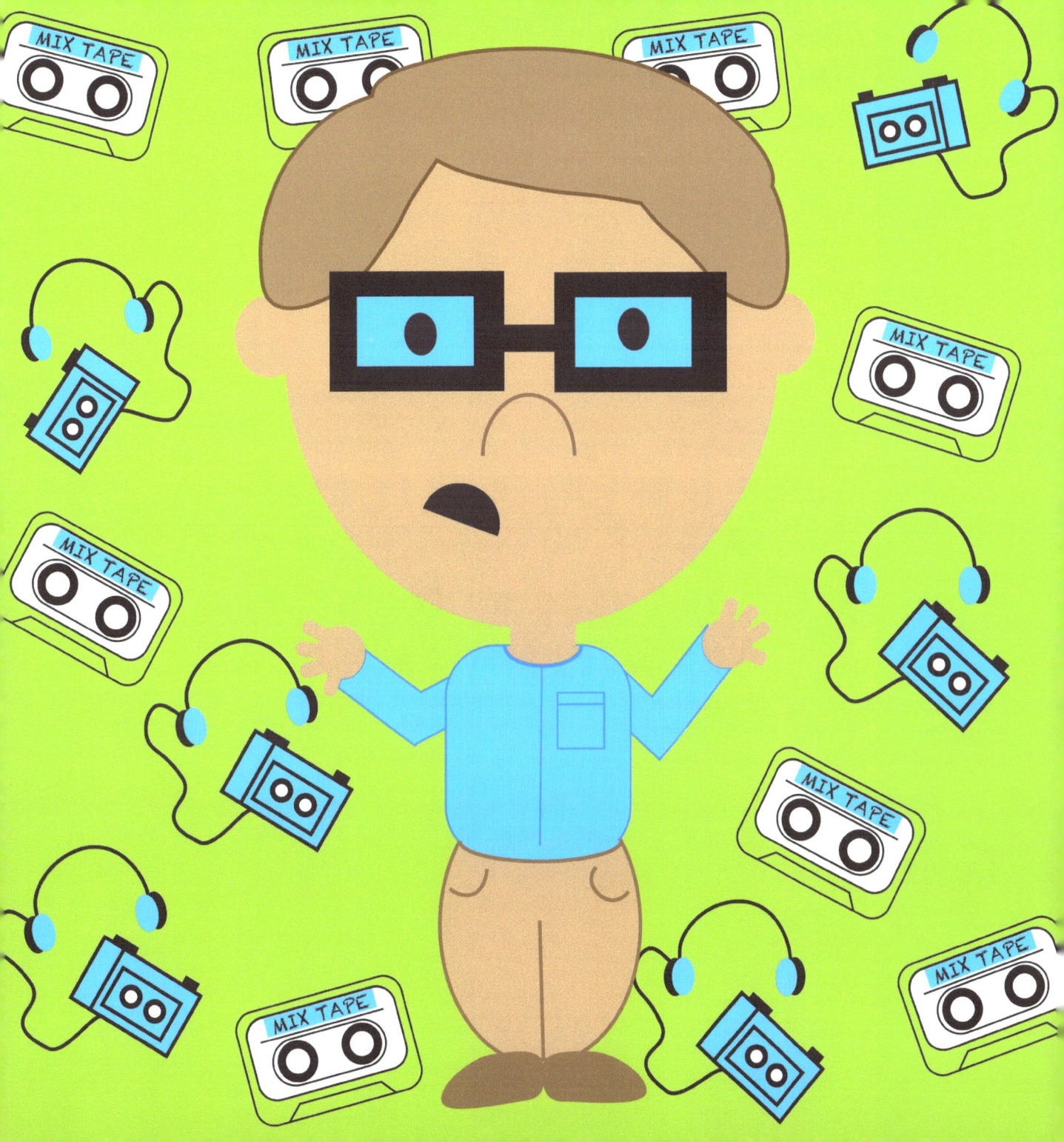

Oh look! Here they are!
A pair that will do!
Not too cheap or too pricey!
And warrantied too!

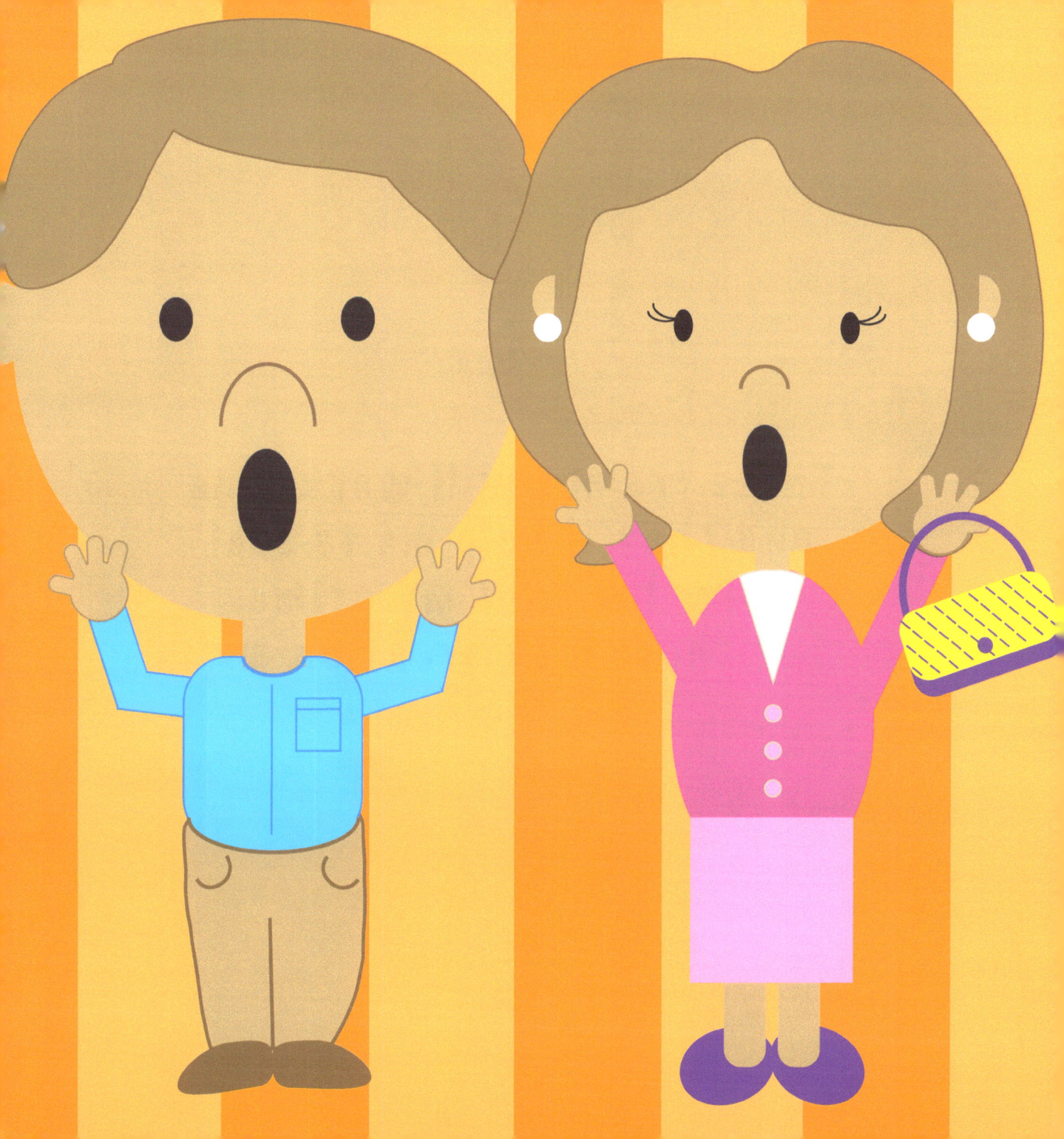

These frames will work fine
and they'll help me to see!
Sure, I'm past my prime,
but these look great on me!

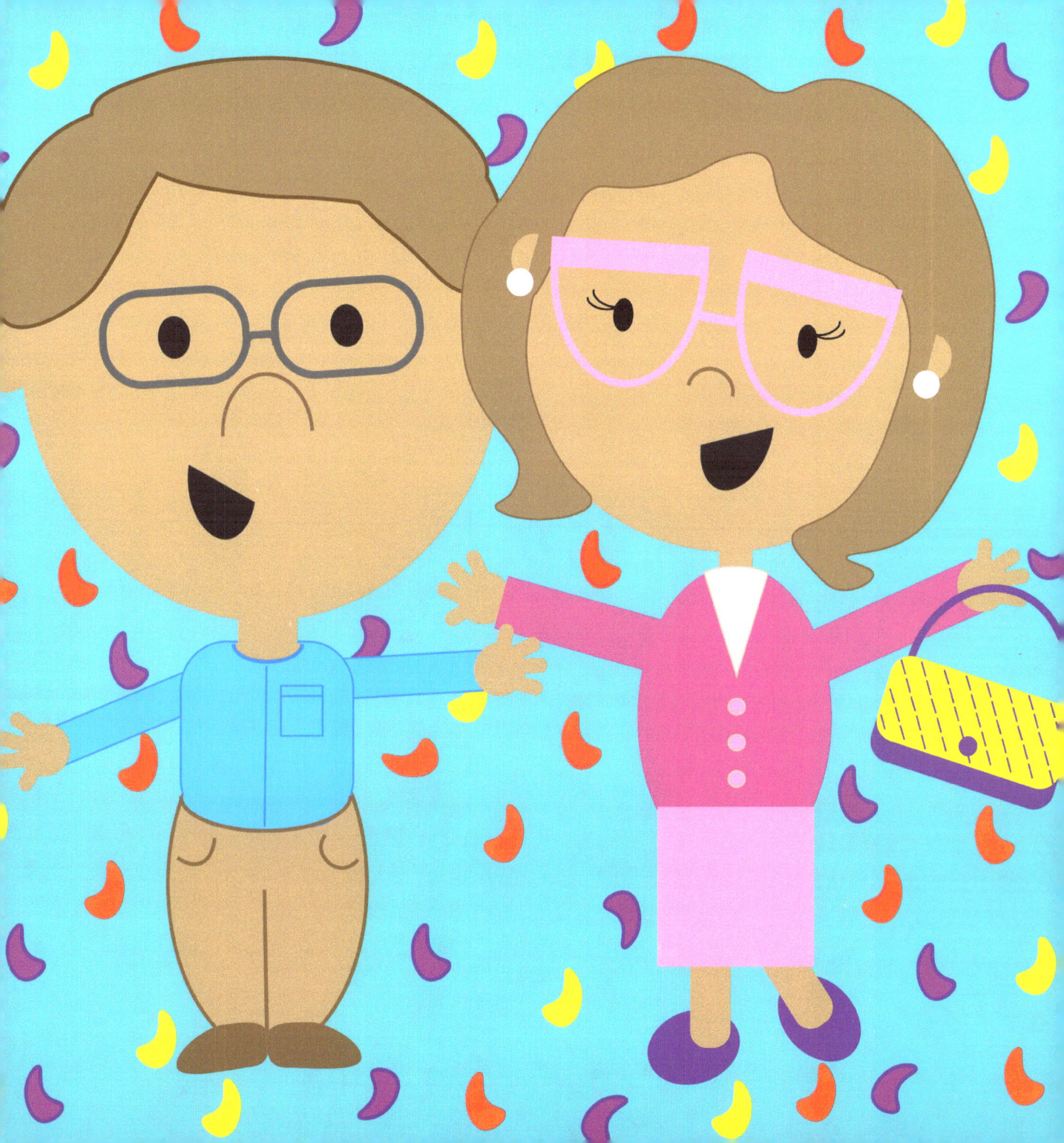

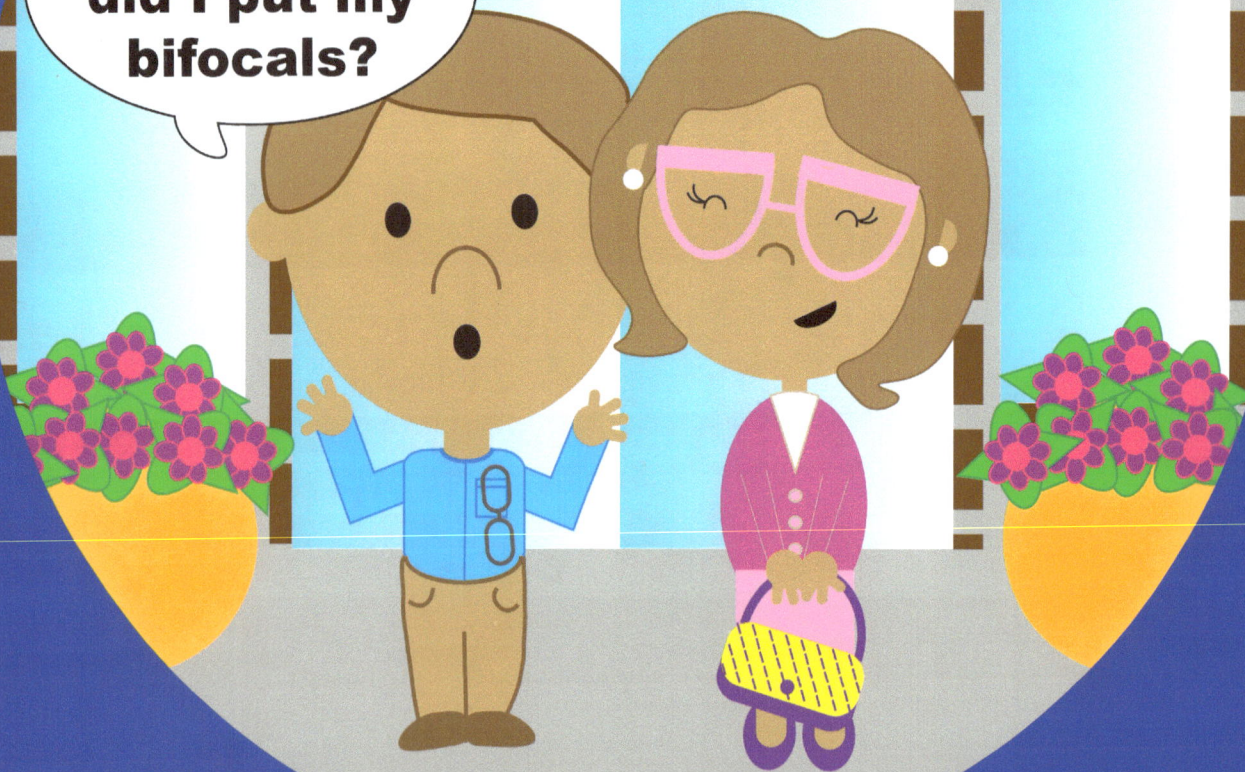

www.ingramcontent.com/pod-product-compliance
Lightning Source LLC
Chambersburg PA
CBHW061149030426
42335CB00003B/164